THE HABIT BLUEPRINT

A EASY-TO-FOLLOW GUIDE FOR LOSING WEIGHT WITHOUT DIETING

Table of Contents

Introduction

Many people want to lose a lot of excess weight. But people are often misinformed, mainly because of the many hyped-up claims and promises of seemingly instant ripped abs and toned butts through severe dietary restrictions. These may come as a result of the kinds of food, total calories, or both and inhumanly difficult exercise routines that are more appropriate for professional athletes and fitness competitors than regular human beings. They believe such hype and go all-out, only to find out the hard and bitter truth that for regular people, such methods aren't only impractical but downright unhealthy.

Losing weight isn't rocket science. It's all about having the right habits and ditching unhealthy ones. In fact, having the right habits can help you effortlessly (or exert minimal effort only) lose weight and keep it off. It will take longer, however, compared to the hyped up promises of many of today's fad crash diets. But make no mistake about it, slower is better when it comes to long-term weight loss and maintenance.

This is what this book is about, i.e., losing weight with minimal effort over the long-term through development of the right weight loss-related habits. Within the pages of this book, you'll learn what habits are, why they're powerful when it comes to accomplishing your desired bodyweight and, more importantly, you'll learn many weight loss habits that can help you lose weight with minimal or no effort and without having to go through dieting and Navy SEAL-like exercise regimens. These habits don't require much effort to develop but, once developed, can synergistically ramp up your long-term weight loss and maintenance.

So, if you're ready, turn the page and let's begin!

The Science behind the Habits

We can think of habits as the behaviors and rituals we automatically carry out. These help us to perform important activities like taking a bath, going to work at a certain time in the morning and even brushing our teeth without even having to think about doing them. Habits help us free a huge chunk of our brains' resources so that it can perform more important and complex activities like figuring out the fastest route to work during rush hour or what gift to give your spouse after forgetting your anniversary.

All of us have many habits that we live out every day, which we can categorize into three types:

1. Habits that we carry out daily without even being conscious of them because they've been part of our daily lives for a very long time. These include brushing our teeth, combing our hair, or using deodorant.
2. Habits that are important and beneficial for us but take conscious effort to establish and maintain like exercising on a regular basis,

sleeping long enough every day and eating certain healthy foods.
3. Habits that are harmful to us like spending more than we earn, eating more than what we can burn on a daily basis and procrastinating.

One of the most intriguing questions ever asked about habits is where in our brain are they stored? Scientists found that a section of the brain called the basal ganglia is responsible for creation and maintenance of habits. And through this discovery, scientists were able to understand how some people continue living out certain habits even after significant injuries to the brain. These habits include being able to find one's way back home despite not having any conscious memory of where they're trying to go. People who have suffered substantial injuries to the brain were still able to access and perform old habits for as long as their brain's basal ganglia remained unscathed. And according to the most recent research on habits, it appears that habits can be so deeply rooted in our brains that even if we no longer benefit from doing them, we can still continue living them out.

A Duke University study demonstrated that more than 40 percent of the things we do every day aren't intentional and conscious but are habitual, i.e., automatic and unconscious. This study's results suggest that by simply replacing old, bad habits with healthy new ones, we can make very significant changes in our lives. And those who are able to understand this idea fully and apply it in their lives are able to discover exciting ways to significantly improve their lives.

The Importance of Habits

If you want to make significant improvements to your health and fitness, you must make healthy living a habit. And crucial to living a healthy life is converting newly-learned healthy living principles, nutritional strategies and physical fitness routines into habits. If you ask successful people about the importance of cultivating the right habits in their personal success, they'd have no difficulty telling you why. But what about you: do you know why it's important for you to be able to cultivate and maintain excellent habits, especially for successfully losing weight and keeping it off?

In case you're not aware of why you'll need to establish excellent habits in your life, here are some very good reasons why you should start establishing them as soon as possible:

1. **You Are Your Habits:** One of the definitions of habits is that they're things

that you do regularly without having to think about or be conscious of. Think about it, how do you tie your shoelaces? How do you drive? To answer these things will probably take you a minute or two to figure out or come up with a coherent answer. Why? It's because you hardly pay attention as you do them. In short, they're automatic and don't require thinking. And because they're automatic, they all add up to becoming who you are right now. So, if you want to become a much better version of yourself, e.g., a slimmer and healthier one, then develop and maintain healthy new habits.

2. **You Have the Power to Change Your Habits**: While it's true that your habits play a huge role in determining who you become and eventually, in shaping your life, it's also true that you have the power to change your habits. While it's not going to be easy breaking old and unhealthy habits, it is possible. It's just like running a full marathon for the first time. Many people think that it's an impossible feat but, after training regularly for many months, and after crossing the finish line, they realize that though it was very challenging, it was possible for them to finish a full marathon.

3. **Right Habits Can Lead to Success**: Rome wasn't built in a day, but the Romans were busy laying bricks by the hour. You can make the case that bricklaying was their foremost habit because that's what they did day in and day out until Rome finally became, well, Rome! Habits are those small bricks that if laid consistently over time accumulate into meaningful accomplishments or successes. If your goal is to lose 40 pounds this year, cultivating and maintaining healthy weight loss habits can help you lose one to two pounds every week. And over the course of several weeks or months, those pounds you lose can accumulate to your target weight loss.

4. **Strong Foundations for Long-Term Success**: Because you eventually become your habits, it follows that establishing the right habits can set the tone for the rest of your life. If you persist with unhealthy eating habits and a sedentary lifestyle, you're setting yourself up for a lifetime of possible sickness and physical weakness. But if you cultivate and maintain healthy eating and physical fitness habits, you're setting yourself up for a lifetime of good health and fitness ahead.

5. **Habits and Optimal Use of Time**: As humans, it's not surprising to find that most of us waste a considerable amount of our time. Human nature dictates that we usually go for the easier stuff with little or no value instead of the challenging and difficult tasks that can make our lives so much better in the long run. By making these difficult and challenging things habits, they can become much easier to do on a regular basis to the point where we can consistently do them within shorter periods of time. When we're able to do that, we can do more important things for the same amount of time, i.e., optimal personal productivity.

6. **Habits Reduce the Need for Motivation**: While motivation is a very powerful tool for getting things done, especially the relatively challenging ones, it's not a very good way to power yourself toward accomplishing your goals. Why? It's because motivation is a fickle or volatile resource, i.e., one day your motivation is high and, on the next day, it may be low or non-existent. Imagine if you relied on something as fickle as that for doing the important things. You'll never be consistent enough to get any meaningful accomplishments. But when you turn those

important things into habits, they become automatic and therefore, consistent. In fact, you might even have to use willpower just to keep yourself from not doing them! The right habits will make it much easier for you to accomplish your goals because you'll be able to consistently do what's necessary for success without exerting much, if any, effort.

Keystone Habits

To successfully lose weight and keep it off even without "dieting," you'll need to develop many small habits that collectively and over the long run can help you accomplish such goals. However, there are two challenges to doing this.

First, your willpower reserves are limited. Therefore, you'll probably have to focus on one or at most, two habits at a time. The only consideration to this approach is the second challenge to this approach, i.e., that it may take much longer for you to get all the important weight loss and weight maintenance habits into the point you may get impatient and quit altogether. If you think about the fact that it may take quite a while to turn an action into a habit, you may find yourself turning impatient.

There is a way to make developing weight loss and maintenance habits a whole lot easier. It's called keystone habits.

Keystone habits are habits that can make it much easier or automatically lead to other habits. Keystone habits set off a chain effect of habit development that can allow you to proverbially hit multiple birds with just one stone. When you think of a long series of dominoes, keystone habits are the first domino, which if toppled automatically leads to the toppling of many other dominoes.

If you focus on keystone habits, you'll be able to use less willpower reserves or self-discipline but develop multiple new habits. A good example of a keystone habit is commuting to work. By making it a habit to take public transportation to and from work every day, you automatically get to develop other good habits like:

1. Regular exercise via long and brisk walks to and from your house, bus stops, subway stations, etc.;
2. Listening to personal productivity podcasts on your way to and from work while on the bus or train; and
3. Saving money through reduced gasoline consumption and vehicle maintenance expenses.

Developing keystone habits can play a crucial role when it comes to achieving your biggest personal and professional goals. Most of the important habits for losing weight and keeping it off without having to "diet" that I'll discuss in the remaining chapters of this book may be considered keystone habits because they can help you automatically develop other healthy habits or at least make it much easier to do so.

Here are some of the most important keystone habits anybody should cultivate for overall success and personal productivity:

Positive Self-Talk

When you develop the habit of talking to yourself in positive ways, one of the automatic changes that will happen is that you greatly reduce your negative self-talk. By focusing on positive internal dialogue, you automatically de-focus or greatly reduce negative self-talk.

Excellence versus Perfectionism

A perfectionist habit is a harmful keystone habit. Why? Not only is perfection impossible to achieve, it also results in:

1. Constant disappointments with one's results regardless if they're great or excellent;
2. Chronic frustrations with one's efforts;
3. Procrastination, i.e., won't proceed to the next steps unless the current ones are perfected; and
4. Burnout.

On the other hand, excellence is a very good keystone habit to develop and maintain. What is excellence? It means doing your best and acknowledging your limits. That means you don't have to wait until you're able to perfectly finish something in order to move on to other things. However, excellence will compel you to give it your best and achieve high quality results, which is possible and beneficial to you and others.

When you focus on excellence, you automatically create new and healthy habits. One is you'll be able to unconsciously reduce (or even eliminate) perfectionism. Another habit that may be borne out of developing the habit of excellence is focusing on one thing at work instead of multi-tasking. Another is the habit of reviewing your work before submission to your bosses or other higher authorities. And all of these consequential habits provide their own sets of benefits that when put together can help you accomplish your goals and dreams much faster than you may have thought possible.

Proactivity

Being proactive means, among other things, taking the initiative to do things without waiting for other people to act first or circumstances to happen first. It also means taking responsibility for the results one gets in life – positive or negative – instead of ascribing them to other people and circumstances.

When you develop the habit of being proactive, you automatically develop other good habits such as:

1. Working on and finishing tasks on time or earlier;
2. Looking for solutions for problems instead of reasons for them; and
3. Doing things regardless of how you feel, how others do their jobs or what the weather's like.

When you become a habitually proactive person, your chances of successfully getting things done and accomplishing your goals become so much higher because you minimize the ability of external and internal circumstances hijacking your efforts and your success.

Saving Money

The habit of saving money can automatically help you develop other good financial habits like:

1. Cutting down on unnecessary expenses;
2. Making and bringing a grocery list every time you go to the supermarket;
3. Planning your weekly, monthly and annual finances
4. Investing; and
5. Monitoring your personal finances by listing down all your expenses and income.

The Habit Loop

The concept of the Habit Loop explains how habits work. Understanding using it is the key to successfully stopping bad habits and developing good ones in their place.

You can think of the habit loop as a neurological one that is responsible for all your habits, regardless if good or bad. This loop has three important elements:

1. The cue;
2. The routine; and
3. The reward.

The extent to which you understand and use these elements is the extent by which you can identify, analyze and replace bad habits with healthy new ones.

The Cue

Habit cues refer to anything that activates a habit, i.e., triggers it. The most common types of cues include:

1. Circumstances;
2. Emotions;
3. Locations;
4. People;
5. Preceding actions; and
6. Times of the day.

For example, you tend to binge eat when you don't eat anything for more than 3 hours after your last meal or you tend to be late for work the following morning whenever you watch your favorite Netflix shows the night before. Advertisers bank on their ability to create advertisements that trigger certain emotions in you to make you buy their products or avail of their services because they understand that emotions can be powerful cues to create habitual buyers.

The cue is a very powerful force when it comes to habits activation. Cues can compel the human brain to automatically execute the habit and to resist the cue requires much effort because of the satisfaction that's often experienced from following cues.

The Routine

You can consider the routine as a habit's most visible element, i.e., it's the behavior that you probably want to stop or replace with something healthier. Or it can be one that you want to reinforce, especially if beneficial.

The Reward

The brain uses rewards as the basis for reinforcing habits, i.e., rewards make habits worth remembering and repeating over and over again. Rewards can be tangible or intangible, depending on the person.

I remember Tony Robbins saying that all of us have two general reasons for behaving the way we do: love of pleasure or fear of pain. Practically everything we do has one or both as rewards.

For example, smokers can't stop the habit because nicotine is an addictive substance that produces pleasure sensations, which is irresistible once a person gets hooked on it. For smokers, the pleasure of nicotine is much more powerful than the fear of acquiring serious sicknesses from smoking, if there's any fear at all.

For people who don't take elevators and who'd rather take the stairs regardless of how many floors they need to climb, the rewards may be:

1. The pleasure of knowing they're doing something good for their heart and the fear of dying from poor cardiovascular health;
2. The fear of being in a closed space and being trapped in it, i.e., claustrophobia; or
3. The pleasure of knowing all other people in the office can't climb ten flights of stairs to the office and only that person can do it.

Disrupting the Habit Loop for Making Habit Changes

You can overcome bad habits and acquire new ones that can help you lose weight without "dieting" by learning how to disrupt the habit loop. Bestselling author of The Power of Habit, Charles Duhigg, recommends a practical but effective way to replace bad habits with new and better ones.

The first step is to identify the routine or the habit. You can easily identify the routine because it's simply the behavior that you wish to replace or get rid of. It may be getting soda from the vending machine after every lunch together with your officemates.

Once you've identified the habit, you can start identifying the cue and the associated rewards for that particular habit. In this particular example, it may be the energy rush or the pleasurable taste of soda after lunch. Or it could be the pleasure of feeling not being left out by your office mates who also drink soda.

The second step is experimenting with the rewards of the habit. Now, rewards are frequently hidden from plain sight, which means you'll probably have to do some thinking or experimenting to find out what those rewards are.

Experimenting with your habits' rewards consumes the most amount of time when it comes to replacing habits. Whenever you feel a strong temptation to go through the routine, consider changing the reward, the routine, or both. Note the changes and don't be afraid to experiment with different theories regarding your routines' drivers.

For example, do you really want the soda or do you just want the company of your friends who happen to drink soda from the vending machine after eating lunch? When you try out a different routine, ask yourself 15 minutes after if you're still craving or looking for the original reward. It might be the reward you're after was really socialization and not the soda.

The next part is isolating the cue, which can be very challenging considering the myriad number of stimuli you're exposed to every single day. Several studies found that most habit cues may fall under any of the following categories:

1. Circumstances;
2. Emotions;
3. Locations;
4. People;
5. Preceding actions; and
6. Times of the day.

To identify your specific habit's possible cue, answer the following questions and write your answers down so that you can look for possible patterns concerning when the temptation to act out the habit arises:

1. Where are you?
2. What time did you start to feel the temptation arise?
3. How are you feeling, i.e., your emotional state?
4. Who is with you?
5. What action or event immediately preceded the temptation or the urge to act out the habit?

Once you've identified your cues or triggers, it's time to plan your strategy to work around or beat the cue. For example, if the need to socialize was the primary need for getting soda after lunch with officemates, a good plan might be to start making it a habit to walk over to an officemate's desk after every one or two hours of work. By doing so, you may be able to satisfy your social interaction cravings and may make it easier for you to not go with them when they get soda after lunch.

How Long Does It Take to Form New Habits?

One of the most prevalent beliefs about habits is that on average, it takes about 21 days or three weeks of continuous execution to form a habit. Is this an accurate belief about the amount of time one can form a new habit?

To answer the question, let's consider the results of a study that was conducted at the University College London. In said study, researchers asked 96 participants to select a daily behavior that they'd like to turn into a habit. All 96 participants chose something they hadn't been doing yet that can be repeated daily.

Many of the habits the participants chose to develop were related to better health like running for 15 minutes after dinner or eating lunch with a piece of fruit. For 84 straight days in which the study was conducted, the participants reported whether or not they performed the habit via a website on a daily basis. They also reported if the behavior felt automatic and if so, how automatic it felt.

Automaticity, i.e., the acting without conscious thinking, appears to be the primary driving force behind habits. And it's also an important factor when answering the question of how long it really takes on average for people to form a new habit.

Based on the study, participants took an average of 66 days to form a new habit. Don't take that 66 as the average or central duration, because it meant it was longer than 66 days for some while for others, it was shorter than 66 days. And the type of habit being formed also played a central part in determining how long the new habit was set.

For example, the subjects who chose to develop the habit of drinking a glass of water immediately after eating breakfast took about 20 days to achieve optimal automaticity, i.e., to make it an automatic habit. Some habits, like doing as much as 50 sit-ups in the morning after drinking coffee took much longer, with one participant still not being able to make it a habit by the time the 84-day study period was concluded. A simpler exercise habit like taking a 10-minute brisk walk after eating breakfast proved to be more achievable, with optimal automaticity being achieved within 50 days for one of the participants.

An interesting observation during the study was that the repetitions that came earlier appeared to be most beneficial when it came to establishing a new habit and over time, the gains from succeeding repetitions declined. As the study's lead proponent explained, developing new habits is similar to running up a steep hill that slowly plateaus as one gets closer to the peak. During the early parts of running such a hill, the rise in elevation with every stride was significant. But as the hill starts plateauing near the top, the increase in elevation with each stride decreases.

For some of the study's participants, the declines in gains were more pronounced. They weren't naturally pre-disposed to forming new habits, with the "speed" at which they developed new habits surprising even the researchers. Using extrapolation of data gleaned from 84 days of the study, it appears that such participants would've taken almost a year – 254 days to be exact – to form new habits.

So, let's go back to our original question: is 21 days enough to form a new habit? Based on this study, the answer is it depends on the habit you want to form. If it's as simple as gulping down a glass of water after eating breakfast every day, then it may be enough. If you're looking to learn new habits that are much harder or complex, it will most likely take much longer than three weeks.

Habits for Weight Loss

In the remaining chapters of this book, we'll talk about habits that, when developed, can help you lose weight even if you don't seriously diet. I've grouped these habits into categories, i.e., mental, eating, lifestyle and social habits. And, as mentioned earlier, many of these may be considered keystone habits, which means developing them can help you build other good habits without breaking much of a sweat.

Mental Habits

I'd consider mental habits as probably the most keystone of keystone habits. Why? It's because the way we think about and our attitude towards life has the most impact in terms of shaping our lives. And this would include losing weight and keeping it off.

When it comes to shedding off excess pounds, experts say that having the right attitude can be very helpful in terms of thinking ourselves thin. According to the author of the bestselling book Fit to Live, Dr. Pamela Peeke, M.D., we must reduce our "mental fat" if we hope to eventually reduce our body fat levels. She recommends taking a close look at our habits and patterns that may be getting in the way of successful weight loss and maintenance.

Every person has an excuse for not changing bad eating and lifestyle habits with good ones or for failing to sustain initial efforts at changing them. There's always a reason for justifying failure like family problems, work issues or other problems. If you want to successfully lose weight, you'll need to change your patterns or routines regardless of your personal challenges or circumstances.

Patience Really Is a Virtue

One significant mental roadblock to successfully losing weight is the desire to lose too much weight too soon. And this desire isn't exactly baseless or unreasonable considering that the Internet and TV is loaded with so many products and services claiming rapid fat loss. Unfortunately, most of them aren't entirely truthful and in fact, many of them overpromise and under-deliver. But most of the public who are desperate to lose weight either ignore the red flags or aren't aware of the absurdity or inaccuracy of the claims made by such products and services' marketers.

The ideal weight loss rate should be two pounds per week at most. More than that runs the risk of water loss or worse, muscle mass loss. And when you lose muscle mass, your metabolism slows down and your weight loss results quickly plateau.

But people today are generally unable to practice delayed gratification – they always want instant results. Regardless if it took them months or years to gain all that excess weight, they want and insist on losing it all in just a few days or weeks. And if you do get to lose so much weight in a few days or weeks, it's probably not going to last because you'll lose more muscle mass than fat. And when that happens, you'll have an even harder time losing weight over the long run, if at all.

Having established the importance of patience when it comes to losing weight, here are some good mental habits to cultivate for losing weight.

Visualization

One of the best ways to "command" your body to lose weight – and keep it off – is to visualize yourself thin regularly. In your mind's eyes, see yourself as losing weight. Imagine how you'd look at least six months down the road and how it must feel to lose those unwanted pounds. If you want to have an easier time visualizing yourself thin, look up some old pictures of you prior to your weight gain. Save a copy on your phone and computer and set them as your wallpaper on both devices o you can frequently see yourself thin.

Think Positively but Realistically

Positive thinking can be such a powerful force for accomplishing goals, including weight loss. If you're a perennial pessimist, it'll be hard for you to do anything worthwhile because you'll think it'll just be a waste of time. But if you cultivate the habit of thinking positively, you can learn to automatically think of solutions instead of limitations, of success instead of failure.

However, there's a flip side to positive thinking too. And that flip side is being unrealistic. When it comes to positive thinking, more isn't necessarily better and there should be a limit to one's positivity. And that limit should be reality.

Regardless of how many people say with conviction that what your mind can conceive your body can achieve, it's simply not true. In fact, it can even be dangerous because putting all your marbles on something that's highly unlikely or impossible to happen can crush all your hopes and make you jaded.

What does it mean to think positively but realistically when it comes to weight loss? It means looking at your current situations and limitations, taking a look at realistic solutions and setting modest weight loss goals. For example, if you haven't lifted a barbell all your life, thinking positively but realistically would mean making it a habit to go to the gym at least twice weekly instead of daily from the get-go. Or if you're 50 pounds overweight and you've accumulated those excess pounds over several years, don't go for severe caloric restriction programs (a.k.a., "diets") hoping to lose five to ten pounds per week when the healthy limit is just two pounds weekly.

Go for Small

By this, I mean set smaller weight loss goals and take smaller steps toward losing weight. By doing so, you can minimize the stress you'll have to go through to lose weight. And when you're able to minimize stress, the easier it can be for you to do things needed to lose weight on a regular basis. And when you're able to do things needed to lose weight on a regular basis, you can more easily (i.e., with minimal stress and hardship) lose weight over the long term. Slow but steady can help you optimize your chances of finishing your weight loss marathon while fast but erratic can do the opposite.

Practice Accountability

No man or woman is an island. Something as challenging as losing a great amount of excess weight will require the support of the people close to you like family and friends. And one of the mental habits you can cultivate that can help you successfully lose weight or achieve any meaningful goal is to be accountable to somebody.

What does that mean? Being accountable means giving another person authority to call you out or even penalize you if you're not able to do what you're supposed to do like lose a target number of pounds every week or exercising a specific number of times every week. And when you're accountable to someone, you can also put yourself in a position where your accountability partner can help you when you're having difficulty doing what you're supposed to do. Studies have shown that dieters who enlist the help of others tend to lose more weight compared to those who don't.

Plan Your Days the Night Before

When you plan your next day's healthy meals and physical exercise the night before, you already win half the battle. Meaningful and consistent weight loss results will only follow after an effective and detailed plan.

Schedule and plan both your eating and exercise strategies, like you would an appointment with your doctor or client. This means taking it seriously and giving it the necessary priority in your daily life. For example, plan the foods you'll need to eat the next day and see if you'll need to bring your own or if it's available in the places you'll be going to the next day. Planning foods to bring is your guaranteed insurance policy that you will not be put in situations where you'll be forced to eat unhealthy foods.

Enjoy Self Rewards

In particular, learn to reward yourself with meaningful things other than food when you meet certain weight-related goals or objectives. These may include half a day at the spa for a deep tissue massage and sauna, watching a live game of your favorite professional sports team or treating yourself to a nice manicure and facial.

When you reward yourself after accomplishing a mini-goal or objective, you get to do two things. First, you motivate yourself to continue doing what you're doing because you can program yourself to look forward to experiencing pleasure after several days or weeks of challenges. Secondly, you recharge your willpower reserves through something pleasurable, giving you renewed energy and strength to do something challenging over and over again in order to accomplish your main goals.

Log What You Eat

Referring again to Charles Duhigg's bestselling book The Power of Habit, he cited a study on a very important weight management keystone habit: food journaling. In said study, subjects who were merely asked to write down all the food they ate – including volume, time and how they felt – on a food journal. At the end of the study, many of the subjects who journal their daily food intake ended up losing meaningful amounts of weight. How?

When they started writing everything they ate, they had the opportunity to see with their own eyes what they were eating, how much they ate and how they felt before and after they ate what they ate. For many of them, simply becoming aware of what they were eating led to automatic changes in their eating habits, e.g., kinds of foods they ate, how much they ate and managing situations that trigger them to eat unhealthily.

When you journal, you may be able to easily change your eating habits through simple awareness, too. That's why food journaling is an important mental keystone habit to develop and maintain if you want to lose weight without "dieting" and keep the weight off.

Eating Habits

Now that we've covered mental habits that can have a huge impact on your weight, it's time to talk about important eating habits that can help you lose weight naturally and keep it off.

Many people think that successfully losing weight always involves exercising 24/7 or severely restricting food choices and amounts. You may be one of them. The good news is that it's not always the case. The fact is you can lose weight naturally without having to diet but by simply adopting several good eating habits. While you may not lose "10 pounds a week" contrary to what many proponents of unhealthy diets are claiming, you can lose 10 pounds over several weeks or months without going through hell and still enjoy life. You can lose a significant amount of weight by simply changing many small habits that may seem inconsequential but can collectively provide meaningful weight loss benefits over the medium to long term.

Fad crash diets are the most popular ways to lose a lot of weight in the short term because many people are so impatient thinking losing excess body fat is as quick as preparing a microwaveable meal. Such diets continue gaining more ground among impatient overweight people because they do work, i.e., they lead to significant weight loss in just a few short days or weeks! At least that's how it looks like.

However, there are three major issues with weight loss from crash diets. The first issue is the kind of weight loss. Weight loss by any other name isn't as healthy. Weight loss can be achieved by losing body fat, muscle mass and water. The kind of weight loss that is optimally healthy is body fat loss. But with crash and severely restrictive diets, most weight loss is only water or worse, involves a great deal of muscle mass. Yes, you can lose a lot of weight in the first few days or couple of weeks, but it's mostly water or muscle mass, which means weight loss from such diets will only be short-lived

What's the matter if you lose water or muscle mass? If you lose water, you'll simply get it back when you drink enough water. And I don't think you should dehydrate yourself just to maintain your "weight loss." That's crazy.

Losing muscle mass is even worse. Why? It's because muscles are the most metabolically active tissues in the body, i.e., it's the type of tissue that burns the most calories. Your metabolism – or the rate at which your body burns calories and body fat – is largely dependent on how much muscle mass you have. So when you have more muscle mass, your metabolism's higher. When you maintain your current muscle mass levels, you maintain your metabolism.

But when you lose significant amounts of muscle, your metabolism slows down, which is the second major issue with crash fad diets. And when your metabolism slows down, your body burns less calories every day. At some point, it slows down to the point you no longer lose weight even while severely cutting food intake. You cut your food intake further and in a couple of weeks, your metabolism slows down even more, leading to another weight loss plateau despite barely eating anymore.

You end up becoming physically weaker and way hungrier over time. At some point, you'll break and start to binge-eat because of the intense feeling of food depravity resulting from severe food restrictions over the last few weeks or months. Then, you'll end up gaining back the weight you lost – and probably more. This is the third major issue with fad crash diets.

That's why when it comes to weight loss, slower is surer. Yes, it may not be as "sexy," or it may feel like eternity but gradually losing weight will give you a higher chance of successfully losing your excess pounds and keep them off. This is because doing so will minimize your risks for feeling deprived and dropping out.

The following are some of the best eating habits to develop that – individually or collectively – can help you naturally lose weight without really "dieting."

Watch Your Portions

You don't have to completely avoid your favorite foods, especially carbohydrates, just to lose weight. Just eat everything in smaller portions. That way, you don't feel deprived, which minimizes your chances of snapping back through binge-eating.

One of the simplest ways to eat the right portions is by eating the following amounts of foods with every meal[1]:

1. A fist-sized portion of carbohydrates;
2. A palm-sized portion of lean protein; and
3. A thumb-sized portion of healthy dietary fat.

---

[1] From Shaun Hadsall's Over 40 Abs Solution and Get Lean in 12 program

Another good and simple guideline to use is:

1. Half of your plate should contain non-starchy vegetables like cabbage and lettuce;
2. One-fourth (1/4) of your plate should contain lean protein; and
3. One-fourth (1/4) of your plate should contain complex carbs like rice.

Lay Your Spoon and Fork Down After Every Bite

The underlying principle here is to slow down your eating. This is because it takes time around 20 minutes – give or take – before your brain senses that your tummy is already full. By putting your spoon and fork down with every bite, you give your brain enough time to pick up how full your tummy's already feeling and minimizes your chances of over-eating.

Slowing down your eating can help you feel full faster, too. This is because you'll be able to fully savor your food's flavors, which may be enough to make you feel satiated even while eating less amount of food.

Drink Water

Water contains no calories. So, it doesn't matter if you drink 10 glasses or 5 glasses.

However, it can help make you feel full. So, you can feel full without taking any calories simply by drinking water.

Often times, what we think is hunger is actually thirst. That's why drinking water frequently throughout the day can help you quell many pseudo-hunger pangs in a calorie-free way. Again, you feel less hungry without taking any calories.

To optimize the natural weight loss effects of drinking water, drink a glass or two of water before every meal. Doing so will help you feel full even before you start eating, which can substantially reduce the amount of food you eat during meals. Less food means less calories, which can lead to natural and easy weight loss over time.

Prepare and Pack Your Own Lunch

When you make this a habit, you enjoy a couple of benefits. First, you'll save more money. Consider the fact that commercially available meals are way more expensive than the ones you can make from the comfort of your own home.

Second, you will be able to eat much healthier. It's because most commercially available meals use a lot of unhealthy ingredients. When you prepare your own meals, you know exactly what goes into them. You wouldn't consciously overdo the salt, sugar or other ingredients that are unhealthy at excess amounts, right? Right! And when you pack your own meals, you eliminate the risks of being forced to settle for unhealthy, calorie-dense and expensive meals from commercial establishments.

But the single biggest benefit, a weight loss-related one at that, is being able to minimize risks for skipping meals and binge-eating as a result of getting so hungry due to skipped meals. When you pack your own lunch, you can always eat on time and avoid skipped meals. And when you always eat on time, you don't get so hungry to the point that you're likely to binge-eat to make up for the meal you missed.

Focus on Eating

When you're multi-tasking while you're eating, you'll most likely eat more than you need to. Why? It's because your mind won't be able to focus on how satiated your tummy already is.

Remember our discussion earlier, i.e., about how long it takes for the brain to pick up that the tummy's already full? When you're watching TV or surfing through Instagram while eating, your brain will be too preoccupied to sense your tummy's signal that it's already full. This can make you effortlessly overeat and gain weight in the long run.

When you focus on eating alone, it'll be easier for your brain to pick up on your tummy's satiety signals. This means you can minimize your chances of eating more than you should, which can help you naturally and effortlessly maintain or even lose weight in the long run.

Eat Breakfast

Contrary to what many who are mindlessly riding on the intermittent fasting bandwagon these days, skipping breakfast can be detrimental to your weight loss efforts. In fact, it can make you effortlessly gain weight in the long run. How?

There's a reason why it's called "breakfast," i.e., it's breaking your overnight fast. Having fasted overnight, you'd probably be hungry in the morning. If you don't eat breakfast, you're skipping meals, which will just make your hunger pangs even stronger. When you choose to skip breakfast and go straight to lunch or early lunch, you'd be so hungry that you'd probably eat a horse. Game over.

Eating a healthy breakfast of complex carbohydrates and protein helps you stabilize your blood sugar levels and ensure steady energy in the morning, which can do wonders in preventing sugar crashes and binge-eating on very unhealthy foods. So, don't mindlessly hop on the breakfast-skipping bandwagon. Make eating breakfast a habit so you minimize your risks for overeating later in the day and gaining weight over the long haul.

Smart Snacking

Snacks are a double-edged sword. On one hand, it can make you gain more weight without noticing it. On the other, it can help you easily and naturally lose weight by helping you keep hunger pangs at bay in between meals so that you don't eat so much every meal, e.g., lunch and dinner.

There are many ways to snack smartly but one of the simplest ways you can make it a healthy habit is just bringing a piece of real fruit with you for snacks like a banana, an apple or an orange. Just stick to one serving and combine it with water and you'll be able to snack smartly in a way that can help you control eating portions and lose weight later on.

Limit Your Cheat Meals

One of the reasons they're called cheat meals is because they're not the norm. As such, it's implied that cheat meals should be occasional. While there's no hard and fast rule about it, I'd say 3 cheat meals per week at most is acceptable. And the best time to schedule them is on weekends.

Why even bother with cheat meals? It's because cheat meals offer several benefits. For one, it helps you satisfy your cravings for your favorite but calorie-dense and/or unhealthy foods. A healthy weight loss diet isn't a perfectly healthy one – no such thing. The occasional cheat meals can help you feel good every once in a while and can give you something to look forward to every week and motivate you in terms of developing and maintaining other healthy eating habits.

Another benefit of occasional cheat meals is that it can keep you from getting bored with eating healthy all the time. If you reach the point of boredom, you might burn out and drop off the healthy eating bandwagon. Then, your natural weight loss efforts can stop or worse, you may start gaining weight when you totally ditch healthy eating habits.

Go for Smaller Plates

When it comes to food plates, there's an interesting phenomenon called the Delboeuf illusion. This illusion makes food placed on smaller dishes appear greater in volume than the same amount of food placed on larger ones. This is because the excess spaces of a larger plate makes the foods placed on it look smaller or less than they are while a smaller plate makes the same amounts of food look bigger because it fills up the entire plate.

Now, how can this help you naturally lose weight? When you eat food on smaller plates, you can trick your brain into thinking you're eating a lot of food, which can make you feel fuller with less food. On the other hand, eating food on large plates will make your brain think you're eating small amounts and may trick you into adding more food to the plate to make it look more filled and make the body feel fuller.

So, stick to smaller plates when eating your meals.

Block the Buffet Table View

If you're eating in a place that has a buffet table, eating your food facing away from the buffet area or table may help you limit or manage your appetite. Many times, we tend to eat more than what we should simply because we see more food on the buffet table and other people going back for seconds, even thirds! So, make it a habit to turn your back on the buffet area.

Stock Up on Veggies

Why are vegetables, especially green leafy non-starchy ones, one of the best foods to eat when trying to lose weight? The single biggest reason is low caloric density.

Caloric density refers to how many calories are packed per unit of volume of a particular food item. This means that a food with higher caloric density has more calories per gram compared to a food with lower caloric density.

A good example of this is a packed cup of lettuce and a packed cup of noodles. A packed cup of lettuce has only 8 calories[2] while a packed cup of noodles has 491 calories[3]! By eating a packed cup of lettuce salad and ditching a packed cup of

---

[2] https://www.healthline.com/health/food-nutrition/romaine-lettuce

[3] https://ndb.nal.usda.gov/ndb/foods/show/16082?fgcd=&manu=&format=&count=&max=25&offset=&sort=defau lt&order=asc&qlookup=16082&ds=&qt=&qp=&qa=&qn=&q=&i ng=

noodles, you save 483 calories! It's an effortless way to cut calories and lose weight!

You can eat as much lettuce as you want and not worry about packing on the pounds. In fact, you can eat to your heart's content and still lose weight because of its very low caloric density. Just make sure you don't go overboard on the salad dressing because some commercially available dressings have high caloric densities. Always check the labels for caloric density.

More than just helping you save on calories, veggies can help you get more phytonutrients, i.e., plant-based nutrients, which can be helpful when it comes to achieving overall health. One of the most important benefits you can get from phytonutrients is anti-oxidants, which can help lower risks for serious diseases like cancer.

Lifestyle Habits

Weight gain isn't just all about eating habits. It's also about lifestyle habits, which can have a profound impact on healthy eating habits, too. Here are some healthy lifestyle habits that when developed or acquired can help you keep your weight down to healthy levels naturally.

Get Enough Sleep

You may be thinking, how on earth is sleeping related to weight gain? Allow me to answer that question.

First, not getting enough sleep will make you feel sluggish and lethargic. In short, it'll make you feel like you lack physical and mental energy for getting things done throughout the day.

When you feel like you need a shot of energy, it's easy to make the mistake of thinking extra calories can compensate for the energy deficit due to lack of sleep. Unfortunately, it doesn't. Eating more rice or bread or donuts won't make you feel more alert or awake.

It may do so within the first few minutes of consuming them, but the subsequent sugar crash will make you feel even more lethargic and sleepy. When you crash, you'll be tempted to get another quick energy fix from sweet or sugary foods, which will just perpetuate a never ending cycle of temporary sugar spikes (high energy) and sugar crashes (low energy and lethargy).

Worse, this can cause you to eat a lot of sugary and high processed, calorie-dense foods like donuts, cookies and energy drinks. This can bump up your calories so much that you won't only lose weight, but you might gain more, too.

Another reason why not getting enough sleep can keep you from losing weight, and may even cause you to gain weight, is a stronger appetite. Sleep can significantly impact your body's production of two appetite-related hormones, leptin and ghrelin.

Considered as appetite hormones, leptin is the hormone that suppresses appetite or signals satiety to the brain while ghrelin is the appetite increasing hormone, i.e., it tells the brain that the body is hungry and needs to eat. When you get enough quality sleep, production of leptin is increased while that of ghrelin is reduced. When you chronically lack sleep, your body produces less leptin and more ghrelin, which can make you feel significantly hungrier than normal and cause you to eat much more food.

Not getting enough sleep can also impact your ability to make sound decisions. In particular, chronic sleep deprivation can dull the activity of your brain's frontal lobe, which is the part responsible for controlling your impulses (binge-eating, anyone?) and decision-making. So, chronic sleep deprivation increases the risks for giving in to impulses to eat unhealthy and calorie-dense foods and making unwise eating decisions, e.g., eating frequency and amount of food.

Also, the brain tends to zone in more on pleasure-producing rewards when you're chronically sleep-deprived. This means it's more inclined to look for pleasure-giving stuff like calorie-rich foods (cakes, sodas, ice cream, etc.) in excess amounts. Getting enough sleep regularly helps minimize the tendency to overeat and eat the wrong kinds of foods in high amounts.

Chronic sleep deprivation doesn't just affect your appetite, but it also impacts your metabolism, i.e., your body's ability to burn calories and body fat. Chronic sleep deprivation causes the body to produce excess cortisol, i.e., the stress hormone. Cortisol tells the body to hold on to calories and body fat in order conserve energy and ensure there's enough of it for survival.

The body starts holding on to more calories and body fat for survival by slowing down metabolism. This can lead to weight loss plateaus or worse, weight gain. Consider that researchers discovered that dieters who reduced their average sleeping hours within a two-week period body fat loss dropped by as much as half even if they consumed the same amount of calories. Worse, said dieters felt weaker, less satisfied with the food they ate – which didn't change – and hungrier.

Lastly, lack of sleep can substantially impact your ability to exercise, whether it's lifting weights at the gym or running outdoors. This is because muscles need sufficient rest and recovery time to perform optimally the next day. Recovery and recuperation happen mostly during sleep.

If you're having difficulty getting enough quality sleep every night, here are some very practical habits you can develop to make getting enough sleep into a habit:

1. One hour before sleeping at night, turn off all your electronic gadgets, i.e., computer, tab, smartphone and TV.
2. Don't work in your bedroom or watch TV in it. Doing so will help reprogram your

mind that the bedroom is for rest and sex only. In time, your mind will start to easily fall into the habit of sleeping and resting every time your head hits the sack.

3. Establish a simple bedtime ritual like taking a warm bath, drinking a cold glass of milk or reading a physical book to relax and wind down. Rituals like these help train your mind to automatically activate the body's sleep mode, which can make it easier for you to fall asleep and get enough sleep at night.

4. Sleep and wake up at the same time every day as much as possible, even on weekends. Doing so will make falling asleep and waking up a habit, which will require minimal or no will power reserves to accomplish.

5. Drink your last cup of coffee at 2 in the afternoon at the latest to give your body enough time to flush out the caffeine from your system. Also, eat your last meal for the day at least 2 hours before bedtime.

6. Sleep in total darkness either by turning off all the lights or wearing an eye mask. Darkness triggers the body's melatonin-production mechanism and light suppresses it. Melatonin is a natural sleep hormone and the extent by which your body's ability to

produce melatonin is the extent by which you can naturally fall asleep and get deep sleep throughout the night.

Daily Meditation

Meditation is the practice of focusing one's attention on one thing for extended periods of time, becoming a more mindful person in the process. A person's attention naturally flows or focuses inward instead of outward during meditation.

How long should you meditate? There's no single standard or benchmark for it, but most people find that meditating for at least 10 minutes per session at least once daily is good enough. If you're new to meditation, even just 10 minutes can seem like an eternity so start with where you are and gradually build up to at least 10 minutes.

Now, what's the relationship between meditation and weight loss? Meditation can help you bring your unconscious and conscious minds into agreement when it comes to choosing the behaviors or habits you need to change and developing new and healthy ones. These habits may include the foods you eat, how much food you eat and exercising.

Remember why we focused on mental habits first? Meditation can help you work up your mind towards successfully unearthing and replacing unhealthy weight-related habits. In particular, meditation can help you become more and more aware of the habits and thinking patterns that need to go and give you motivation and mental energy to replace them with much better ones.

Making meditation a habit can also help you stay conscious of your weight loss goals. By meditating regularly, you can put such goals at the forefront of your mind so that you won't forget it and you can continue hacking at it until you succeed.

Another way by which regular meditation can help you lose weight is by improving psychological well-being, particularly by helping you become more mindful. If you recall, many people gain weight and fail to lose weight because of emotional eating that triggers frequent binge-eating. The more mindful you become, the less emotional you become, which means your emotions' power over your appetite becomes substantially weaker over time. At some point, may be able to overcome your tendency to over or binge-eat, which means you can eat less naturally and lose weight.

How do you actually practice meditation? Well, there are a myriad number of ways to do so but here's a very simple but effective way to meditate, which is called the box-breathing technique. It's a breathing meditation technique popularized by bestselling author Mark Divine in his book The Way of the SEAL. Here's how to do the box-breathing meditation:

1. Sit comfortably upright on a back-supported chair.
2. Set your timer for at least 10 minutes.
3. Put your hands on your lap.
4. Close your eyes.
5. Start the breathing cycle by inhaling deeply through the nose for five seconds.
6. Hold your breath for five seconds.
7. Exhale everything through the nose for five seconds.
8. Hold your breath for another five seconds, which concludes one breath cycle.
9. Repeat the breath cycle multiple times until your timer goes off.

The best time to do the box-breathing meditation technique is in the morning when the probability of being disturbed or distracted by other people in your house is at its lowest.

Regular Exercise

At the end of the day, weight loss is all about energy balance or calorie balance. It means that when you consume more calories than what you burn daily, you'll be in a constant state of caloric surplus and gain weight. When you consume less than what you burn daily, you'll be in a constant state of caloric deficit and lose weight. If equal, you'll maintain your current weight.

To lose weight, you can either reduce your caloric intake, increase the calories you burn daily, or both. All of the habits we discussed so far address the reduced caloric intake part. Regular exercise is a habit that addresses the calorie-burning part.

The more you move, the more calories you burn. It's that simple. Two people with the same weight, muscle mass and metabolism will lose different amounts of weight if one doesn't exercise and if the other does.

How much regular exercise do you need? Most experts suggest that 30 minutes of regular exercise at least thrice weekly can help in weight loss. You don't need to train like a professional athlete to enjoy the weight loss and weight maintenance benefits of regular exercise. Brisk walking for 30 minutes thrice a week can be good enough at the beginning, especially if you've been living a sedentary lifestyle ever since. But if you're already fairly active, you might need higher intensity and duration exercises like running or lifting weights. The important thing is you exercise for 30 minutes at least thrice weekly at mid or medium intensity.

So, how do you measure or estimate your exercise intensity level? You can use the talk test to do that. After a few minutes of continuous exercise, try talking as if you're having a conversation with somebody. If:

1. You can carry a normal conversation without any breathing strain like you're catching up with a friend in a coffee shop, your exercise intensity is low;
2. You can barely talk because you have to catch your breath, your exercising at high intensity level; and
3. You can carry a normal conversation albeit with some breathing strain, you're exercising at mid or medium intensity level, which is the ideal intensity level for most people.

Social Habits

Finally, how you interact with other people in social settings can also have a profound impact in your ability to lose or maintain your ideal weight. Here are some social habits that are worth cultivating or need to be replaced with healthier ones.

Clubbing or Bar Hopping

Every once in a while, there's nothing wrong with clubbing or bar hopping. But if this is habitual, it can wreak havoc on your weight loss or weight maintenance efforts.

One reason for this is alcoholic drinks. Many of the drinks in bars and clubs, especially beer, have very high sugar content and therefore, high caloric content. It can be very easy to fall into the temptation of drinking one shot, glass or bottle too many and pile on excess calories when clubbing or bar hopping. That's why if this is habitual, it's best to think twice about keeping this habit especially if you're concerned with your weight.

Join Health and Fitness-Focused Groups

You can have a much easier time sticking to your weight loss plan or endeavors when you know you're doing it with other people. That's why joining and regularly participating in activities of health and fitness-focused groups can do wonders in terms of motivation and support, especially during times when temptations to ditch healthy weight loss habits are very strong.

Where can you join such groups? Local gyms, yoga studios, running clubs and online forums and social media groups are just some of the many places where you can meet and interact regularly with like-minded people with the same health and fitness goals as you have. Your weight loss journey doesn't have to be a lonely one. Joining other people on the same journey can make the journey more pleasant, joyful and easier.

Conclusion

Thanks for buying this book. I hope that through this, you learned a lot about how habits are key to successful weight loss and more importantly, I hope you learned many new habits that can help you lose weight naturally without having to subject yourself to severe and unrealistic diets.

But knowing is only half the battle for losing weight. Action – or application of knowledge – is the other important half. That's why I'd like to strongly encourage you to start applying at least one or two lessons, i.e., establishing one or two habits presented in this book. When you've gotten them down to pat already, then start adding one or two more. Over time, you can incorporate most if not all of the habits in this book in your life and enjoy their synergistic weight-loss benefits without even feeling deprived or weak due to severe caloric restrictions, which many of today's most popular diets do.

Here's to your weight loss success my friend! Cheers!

Reference: None, I'm very familiar with the topic.